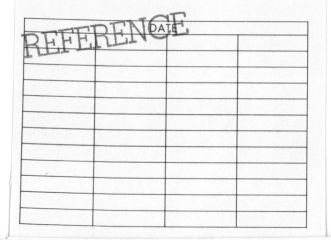

FORM 125 M

cop. 1   SOCIAL SCIENCES AND HISTORY DIVISION

The Chicago Public Library

JAN 19 1979

Received _____

© THE BAKER & TAYLOR CO.

Individual Tactics in Water Polo

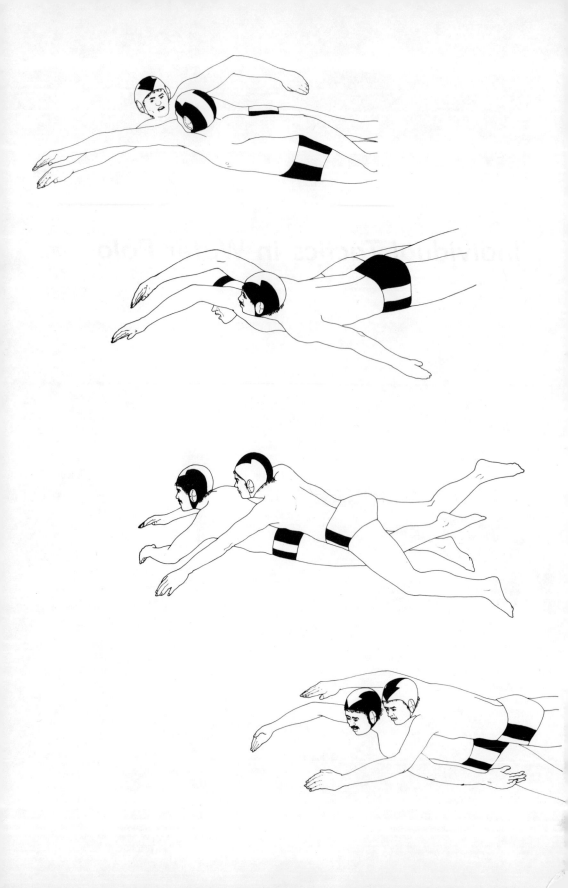

Individual Tactics in Water Polo

James S. Wiltens

Water Polo Coach, Simon Fraser University

Illustrations by William Schuss

Audio Visual Department, S.F.U.

SOUTH BRUNSWICK AND NEW YORK: A. S. BARNES AND COMPANY

LONDON: THOMAS YOSELOFF LTD

© 1978 by A. S. Barnes and Co., Inc.

A. S. Barnes and Co., Inc.
Cranbury, New Jersey 08512

Thomas Yoseloff Ltd
Magdalen House
136-148 Tooley Street
London SE1 2TT, England

Library of Congress Cataloging in Publication Data

Wiltens, Jim 1949-
   Individual tactics in water polo.

   Includes index.
   1. Water polo. I. Title.
GV839.W54   1978 797.2'5 76-50218
ISBN 0-498-02002-9

PRINTED IN THE UNITED STATES OF AMERICA

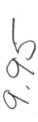

To Mr. Hepner who gave me a love for the sport,
Art Lambert who taught me the game,
and Dr. Martin Hendy whose support and editorial assistance helped
make this book possible.

Contents

Preface

As time has passed, the game of water polo has matured. In the early days you had to be a hairy behemoth, not necessarily a competent swimmer, but you should have known, as one old timer put it, "the art of the boa constrictor caress." Players would leap and run along the bottom of the pool, tackling, punching, gouging, and strangling one another to get a goal. The development of a set of rules and the use of all-deep-water pools phased out water football, and water polo developed into a sophisticated game involving strategy and skill. Both knowledge and proficiency are now required if you want to be an all-star player. It is unfortunate though that many players still play jungle ball: hitting, slashing, and in general committing blatant fouls for which they are penalized by the referee. These players lack the "style" associated with top-caliber individuals.

But what exactly is that ingredient we call *style?* Part of it is experience, another part knowledge, and finally knowing when to attempt a move — timing. Players who have a good coach will probably be well versed in game patterns, but too many coaches ignore teaching individual movements, relying solely on game patterns. This is like giving a soldier the battle plan but forgetting to supply him with ammunition. If your coach does not teach individual movements it is not likely that other competent players will. Often when a player discovers a move he guards it with a certain degree of secrecy and jealousy. When a move is performed on you it usually happens so fast that you rarely get a clear picture of what happened, and it may take years of trial and error before you learn the move.

This book is a culmination of twelve years of watching, analyzing, and performing individual movements and techniques. You will note that the following pages take a rather clandestine approach in that many of the moves described are actually skillful fouls. You don't have to play water polo long at a high school — not to mention the national or international — level to learn that fouling is part of the game; so don't be too self-righteous in this iceberg sport where fifty percent of the action is underwater. The important thing is to avoid blatant fouls and resort to skillful finesse.

As a coach I have taught these moves in what is known as a *cate,* a sequential form of teaching derived from the martial arts. Each move has been broken down into its simplest components, which the player memorizes and performs in his mind, visualizing each movement, body motion, and hand position. After meditating (*Psychocybernetics* by Maxwell Maltz) through a move the player performs it and is criticized. Next we have a dummy opponent who offers no resistance as the move is performed repetitiously. With time, the resistance increases and is at its peak in scrimmage situations. This technique of teaching, along with a clear format-outline of the move, can accelerate player proficiency, cramming years of trial and error into months. Here I want to stress the importance of the player understanding exactly what he is doing. Too many coaches give tremendous instructions like "stick the ball in the cage," "just shoot harder," or, as frustration sets in, "kill the guy." Remember that if the coach is a good teacher the player will understand a move in its entirety and become his own critic and coach—something many coaches are hesitant to encourage.

How To Use This Book

Each move begins with a description of the particular circumstances or situations in which the movement is most useful. The move is then broken down into individual steps explaining exactly what the player is to do.

After reading one or several steps you will come to a diagram that may either illustrate one particular aspect of a move or demonstrate the entire sequence up to that point. Note, in the drawings, that the person performing the move is wearing a dark swim suit. His cap is also dark with a white arrow, and he always has a moustache. The player on whom the "move is being performed" has a white swim suit, a white cap with a black arrow, and is clean shaven.

At the end of the explanation is a memory aid containing key words. When the player is in the water, and learning, the memory aid can help him perform all parts of a move.

At the end of every move there is a table, pointing out possible problems, the error involved, and how to correct those errors.

After becoming proficient at several moves, link them into a sequence such that if you miss the first move you immediately try for another. Combinations of moves are unbelievably potent when performed one after another and distinguish the pro. Here is a chance for you to be creative.

Individual Tactics in Water Polo

1 Moves for Offensive Drivers

SLIP

This move will place you in front of your opponent when you are originally swimming side by side. It is also useful when you want to draw a foul on your opponent.

1. Swim side by side with your opponent, if possible a little ahead.

2. Time your stroke so that it is out of cycle with his (ie., your hand nearest him enters the water as his comes out).

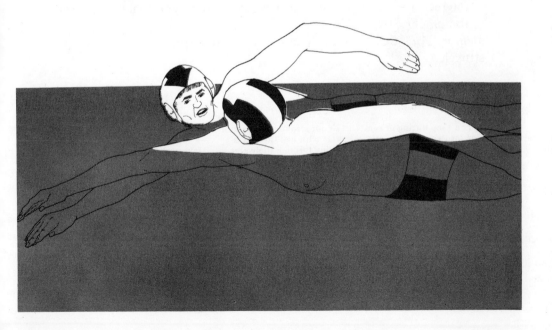

3. Dip your near shoulder to the side and under his upraised arm, sweeping with your near hand to slip your body under and ahead of his.

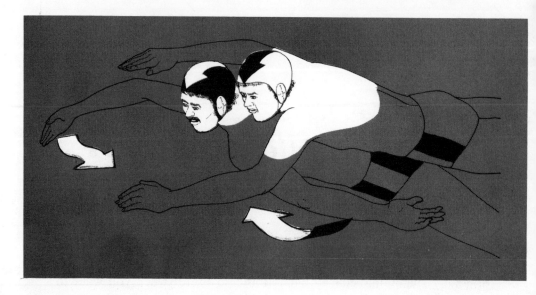

4. Sweeping your hand across the front of your body has placed you in front of him. Now modify your stroke to a rapid dog paddle, trying to lift your arms and draw the foul.

5. If done smoothly and not directly under the scrutiny of the referee, it looks as if the man has swum up on your back, a kick-out foul under FINA rules.

Memory Aid: Stroke out of phase — slip under upraised arm — sweep — struggle.

PROBLEM	CAUSE	CORRECTION
1. You keep hitting or running into your opponent's arm, which prevents the slip.	1. Your stroke is not out of cycle with his. His arm is pulling through the water as you go for the slip.	1. Get your stroke out of phase by speeding up or slowing down. Make sure his near arm is lifting out of the water as you go for the move.
2. He's still at your side after the slip.	2. Either not enough dip with your shoulder, you're not close enough to him to make the move, or you haven't swept with your hand.	2. Close in on opponent, almost rubbing his shoulder, sweep your hand forcefully across the front of your body, pushing you under opponent.
3. Opponent slides all over you in an obvious foul, but no foul is called.	3. Referee has not noticed.	3. Make noise and struggle to start your crawl stroke. Resort to dog paddle if necessary to keep your position in front of guard.

16

FINESSE

The finesse is used to place you in front of the man with whom you are swimming. Usually your opponent is faster than you and an edge is needed. This tactic is most effective at halfway when the referee is not looking.

1. Close in on the opposing swimmer until you are shoulder to shoulder with him. The closer the better.

2. Time your stroke to his such that your arm cycle is slightly behind his. The palm of your hand should be near his wrist.

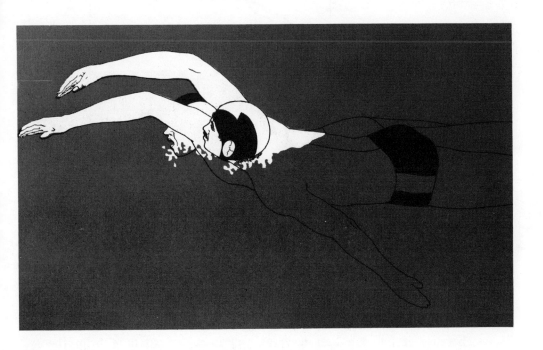

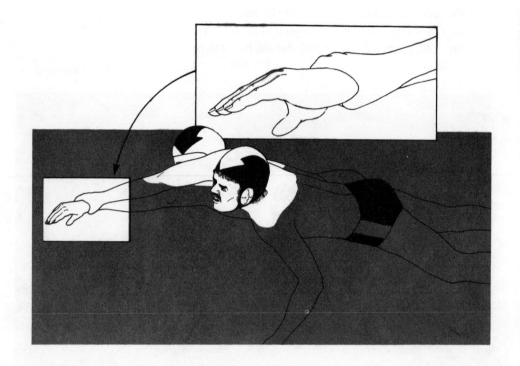

3. As his hand enters the water you should grab his wrist, — his wrist because it has the best leverage and is easiest to hide from the referee.

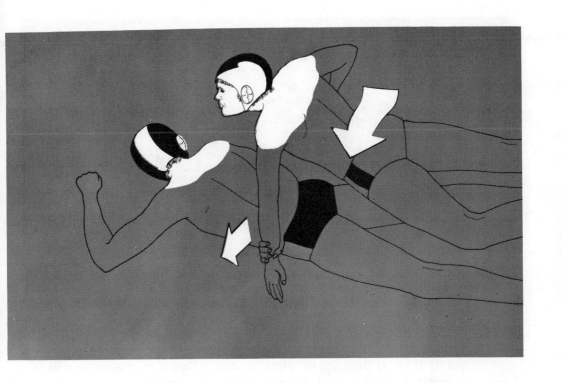

4. Holding his wrist, thrust your hand to the lower middle of your back.

5. Now lower your shoulder and slide under his arm such that he is directly behind you. Release his hand.

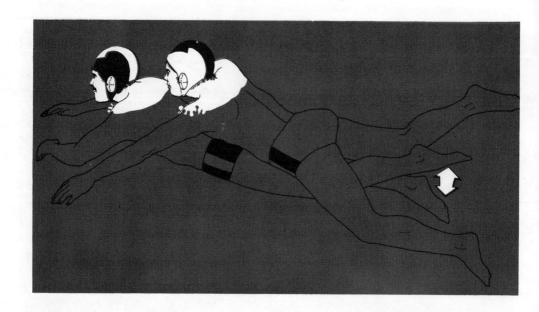

6. Struggle to get your stroke going. You may have to resort to dog paddle if he is high up on your back. (If this is necessary he will probably be called for fouling.) Try to keep your forward momentum.

7. The player is now situated behind you, and the only way for him to get around you is to foul.

Memory Aid: Synchronize — wrist grab — pull across back — slide — struggle.

PROBLEM	CAUSE	CORRECTION
1. Opponent remains at your side after the move rather than behind you.	1. When you grab his wrist you are pushing it down or to your side.	1. When you grab, push his arm across and to the middle of your back.
2. Even when you push the opponent's arm to the middle of your back he remains at your side.	2. You are not sliding under the arm.	2. As you push the arm to the middle of your back, tilt your shoulder down and slip under your opponent.
3. Referee often calls you for fouling.	3. You are grabbing the wrist before it enters the water or you are grabbing too high up on his arm where it is obvious to the referee.	3. Grab the wrist as it enters the water.
4. Can't seem to get his wrist.	4. You probably are not synchronized to his stroke.	4. Slow down or speed up so that your arm nearest the opponent is shadowing his nearest arm.
5. Referee calls you for diving.	5. You are performing the move directly under the scrutiny of the referee.	5. Take a glance at the referee to make sure he is not looking directly at you, then perform the move.
6. You make a beautiful move, but opponent goes right over you.	6. If you could maintain the opponent on your back longer the referee would see the foul. You have probably stopped moving forward.	6. Struggle to keep going forward and make some noise.

CROSS-CHECK BLOCK

When your guard is aware that you are trying to get by him the cross-check is an effective way to take him by surprise.

1. Swim shoulder to shoulder with your guard.

2. Time your stroke so that it is in cycle with your opponents (i.e., your hand nearest him lifts out of the water at the same time as his near hand).

3. If he is swimming next to your right side the move proceeds as follows: As his left hand finishes pulling underwater and is coming out, reach with your left arm across and under his body. You are using your own body to hide your reaching arm from the referee.

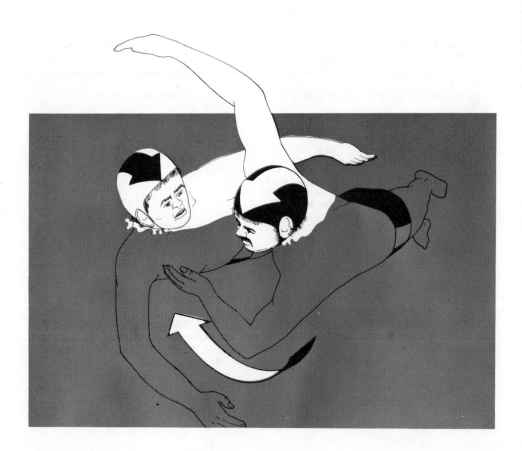

4. Place your left hand against his chest and sweep back, forcing him behind you.

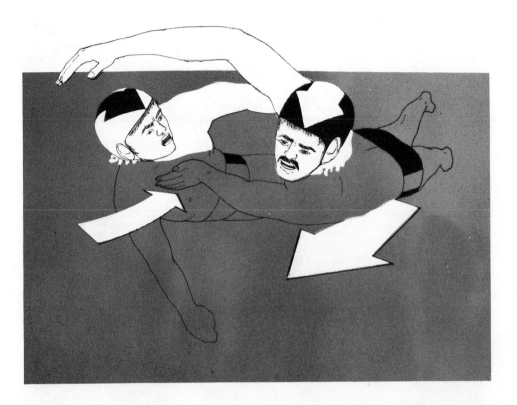

Memory Aid: Stroke in cycle — reach across — sweep.

PROBLEM	CAUSE	CORRECTION
1. Repeatedly called for fouling.	1. Several possibilities: a) you are reaching up on opponent's shoulder or around his neck; b) you are rolling onto your back as you sweep.	1. a) Keep your hand on his chest just below his shoulder. b) If you roll to your back you expose the fouling arm to the referee. Stay on your stomach throughout the move.
2. Hand keeps slipping off of guard's chest, and you have an ineffectual push.	2. Hand is too low on his chest.	2. Place your hand just below his shoulder.
3. You push but it hardly effects his forward momentum.	3. You have not reached all the way across his chest.	3. You should place your hand all the way to the other side of his chest, not the near side.

FORWARD WRIST GRAB

Your opponent is blocking you from driving and is facing you.
1. Face your opponent, hips high and ready to go.
2. In a quick motion, reach with your same hand (i.e., right hand to his right hand, and grasp his wrist).

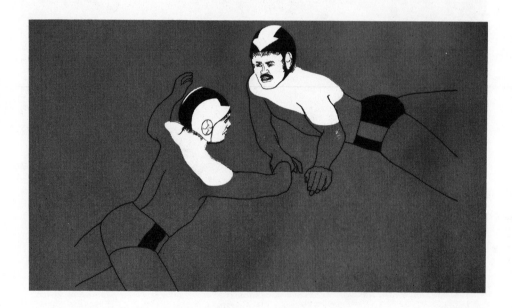

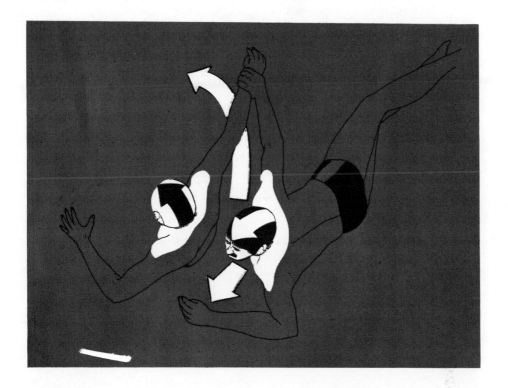

3. Pull his arm around in a circular motion so that his back is turned towards you. This is general for all forward wrist grabs; pull until the opponent's back is to you, — his most vulnerable position.

4. As you start swimming past your opponent, slide so that he is directly behind you and not at your side.

5. You will probably find that you do not have to pull very hard, as his first reaction, when grabbed, will be to pull away. You just have to hold on and direct his action.

Memory Aid: Face him — grab opposite hand — circle pull — slide.

PROBLEM	CAUSE	CORRECTION
1. Player smashes into you preventing the move.	1. You are pulling the opponent directly into you.	1. Pull his arm around in a circular motion away from you.
2. After the move, you find your opponent swimming shoulder to shoulder with you.	2. You have not slipped in behind your opponent after you passed him.	2. After pulling by opponent make a sharp angle to place him directly behind you.
3. You grab his wrist and he in turn uses that hand to grab your wrist as if you were shaking hands.	3. You have reached for the inside of his wrist, his palm facing your wrist.	3. Grab his wrist from the top.
4. You have turned your opponent so that his back is to you, but he continues to spin and hits you in the face with his elbow.	4. You have your head down in the water.	4. He has made a good counter move. Never put your head down or you won't see the elbow coming and have time to avoid it.

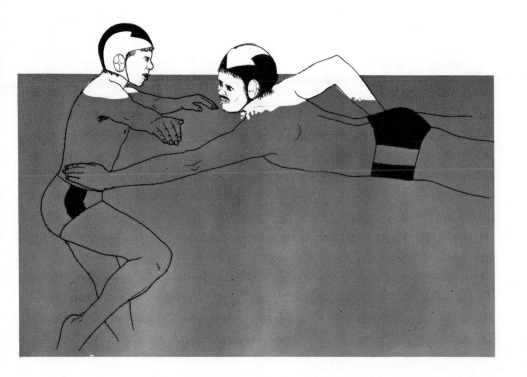

HIP ROLL

This maneuver comes about when your opponent has made the mistake of dropping his hips while facing you.

1. Face your opponent less than an arm's length away. You recognize that he has made an error by letting his hips down.

2. Thrust your arm underwater towards his hip.

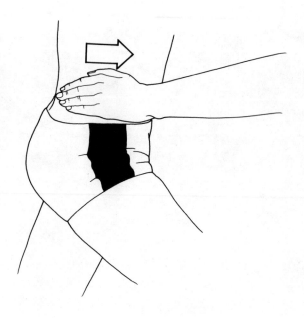

3. Place your hand low on his hip; don't grasp but cup.
4. Pull his hip toward you; don't push down as this is an obvious foul.

5. As you are pulling, start a roll to your back, outside of his arm. Try to stay as close to your opponent as possible while rolling, otherwise you lose leverage.

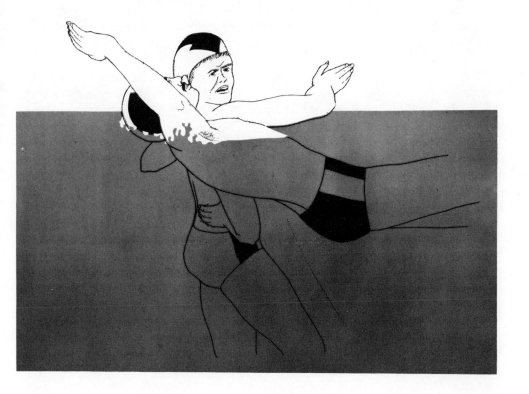

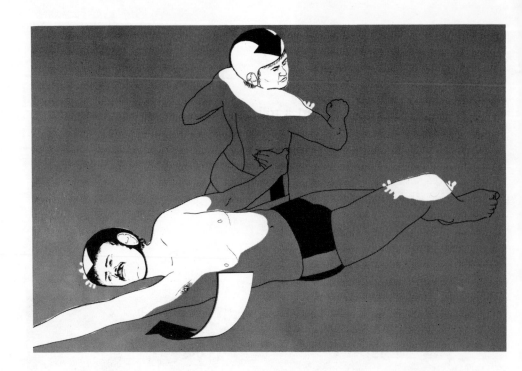

6. As you pass your opponent's body, continue your roll and end on your stomach in crawl position.

7. End the move by sliding to the side such that your opponent is behind you, preferably on your legs.

Memory Aid: Hand to hip — pull towards you — roll close — freestyle — slide.

Variation: Grab his near hand (i.e., your right to his left, and pull as you roll).

PROBLEM	CAUSE	CORRECTION
1. Can't seem to get his hip.	1. He has not made the mistake on which this move is dependent.	1. His hips are not down and he's not ready for the move.
2. Referee calls you for sinking your opponent.	2. You are pushing down on the hip.	2. Pull the hip towards you.
3. Opponent is at your side after the move.	3. You are pushing the man away.	3. Try to stay as close to the man as possible throughout the move.

GRAND FAKE

This is a grandstander's move and requires exceptional timing. The grand fake may be very helpful if you are in the last moments of play and desperately require a goal.

1. The situation is such that you are facing the cage with a potential, though poor, shot. Your defensive man is in front of you.

2. Do a powerful egg-beater, using the hand that is not holding the ball for support. You must convince the man guarding you that you're about to shoot. Charm him with the ball as a snake would charm a bird.

3. We will assume you are right-handed and on a center line with the cage.

4. Pump the ball as if you are taking a shot at the right side of the cage. Bring the ball close enough to the guard to tempt him to lunge for the ball. If he lunges, your move starts.

5. Carry the ball away from his lunge, rotating your body around 360 degrees.

6. As you spin, lunge forward, which should put the defensive man at your side. Place the ball in front of you, no more than an arm's length away, and drive at the cage.

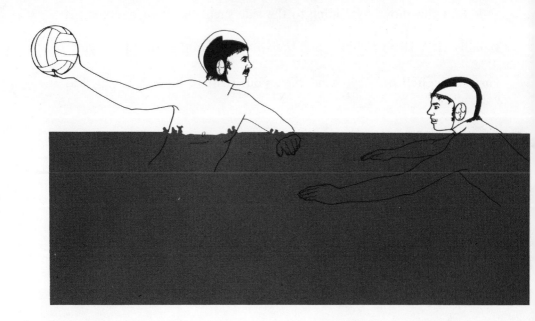

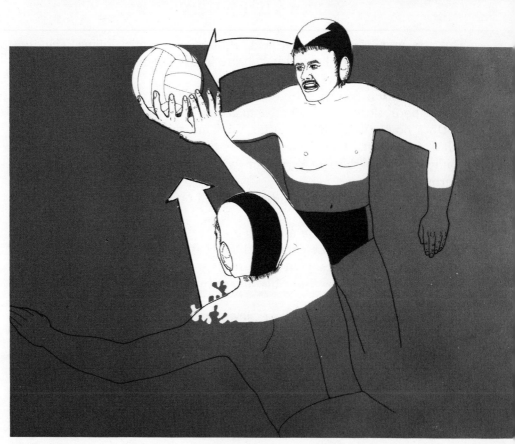

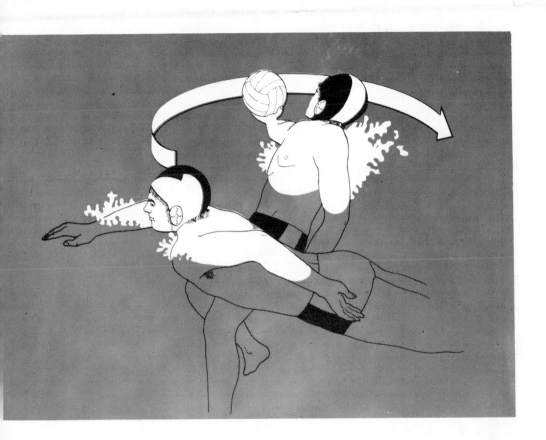

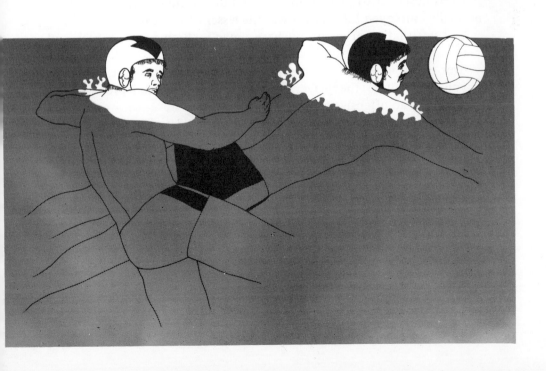

7. This maneuver should only be attempted when you have open water in front of you after the move. Don't do it if you will swim into more defensive players.

Memory Aid: Fake shot — tempt — 360 degree spin — place ball — drive.

PROBLEM	CAUSE	CORRECTION
1. After the spin, you swim right into the defensive man.	1. He has not committed himself by lunging for the ball.	1. The fake shot must be more tempting, waiting long enough for him to lunge for the ball.
2. You can't control the ball as you spin and it falls off your hand.	2. Hand is held flat as you carry the ball around. When you come to an abrupt stop at the end of your spin the momentum carries the ball off your hand.	2. As you complete your spin rotate your hand up behind ball to brake the force.
3. You lose the ball to your opponent after completing the spin.	3. You have thrown the ball in front of you after spin, giving opponent a chance to get it.	3. Place the ball less than an arm's length in front of your face. You should be able to retrieve it if any difficulty arises.
4. Ball is knocked out of your hand during the spin.	4. Ball is held near your head.	4. Hold ball at full-arm's length throughout spin.

HAMMER

I was hesistant to include this move, but considering the alternatives normally employed I decided it was the lesser of two evils.

1. The situation often arises where a man is chasing at your heels and trying to grab your ankles. Many players respond to this by rolling over or stopping and kicking the chaser in the head. This is stupid, as you may injure the player, destroy your drive, and probably get called for an offensive foul.

2. The better thing to do is as follows: As the player grabbing at your ankles gets closer, increase your arm turnover, but let your hands slip through the water a little so that you slow down for a moment.

3. During the hesitation the chaser should swim directly into your legs. Just before this happens increase your flutter kick so it is high out of the water.

4. Now come down with the top of your foot against his shoulder and push down hard. This should drive you forward and leave him eating water.

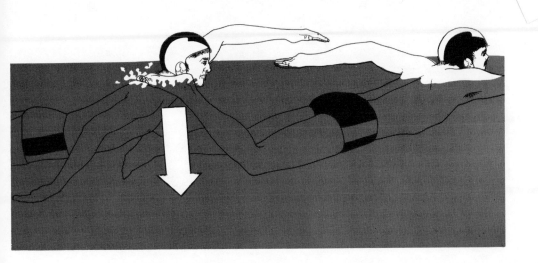

PROBLEM	CAUSE	CORRECTION
1. You get called for fouling.	1. There are a number of possibilities: a) you are kicking much too high; b) you stop dead in the water and come down on him with your kick; c) you roll to your back to kick.	1. a) Kick just high enough to get your foot on his shoulder. b) You should slow down a little, not come to a dead stop. This is accomplished by slipping your hands through the water. c) Stay on your stomach.
2. You hesitate, but the man, instead of swimming into your legs, catches up with you.	2. He is not directly behind you.	2. You must weave back and forth to keep him on your heels.
3. He holds your heels down and you can't get your feet up on his shoulder.	3. He's pushing your feet down with his forearm.	3. Accelerate your kick sooner.

2 Shots

CORK-SCREW SHOT

This shot is used when you are being closely pursued and do not have time to pick up the ball.

1. You have possession of the ball and are swimming at the opponent's cage. Your guard is swimming next to you, at or near your hips.

2. You must be able to reach the four-meter line, preferably on a center line with the cage. The four-meter to three-meter region is ideal for shooting.

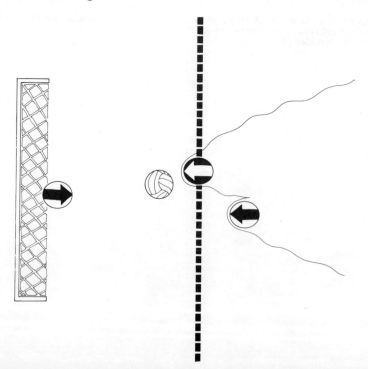

3. As you approach the cage increase the tempo of your flutter kick. This helps to maintain your momentum and high position in the water during the shot.

4. Take shorter strokes and increase the rate of turnover. Increased turnover will keep your shooting hand near the ball longer than a lengthy pull.

5. Be a little sloppy on your hand entry to set up some splash. This helps to confuse the goalie and camouflage your coming shot. Some players shoot through a virtual curtain of water.

6. Now for the shot. If you are right-handed, make your normal hand entry but, instead of stroking, rotate your arm so the ball is resting on your fingertips.

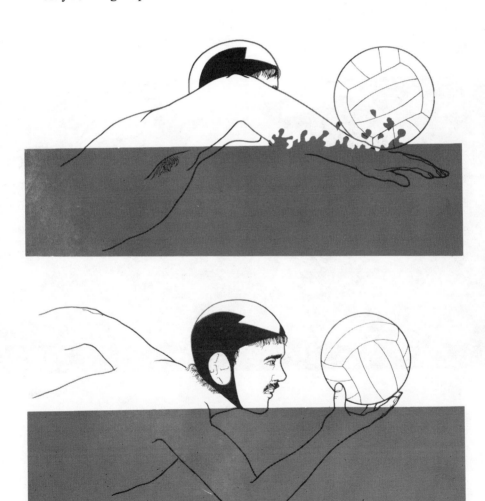

7. Next, cock the ball. This is done by retracting your arm until the ball is near the side of your head. Your hand remains under the ball the whole time.

8. To shoot the ball, thrust your hand forward in a cork-screwing motion. Started properly, your palm will be facing the ceiling under the ball at the start of the shot. As your hand travels forward your palm goes around 180 degrees, such that your palm is facing the water at the end of the shot.

9. Throughout the progress of the shot you must continue to swim with your non-shooting arm (i.e., from the moment you pick up the ball with your right hand your left should make one complete stroke revolution, finishing the stroke as the ball leaves your hand).

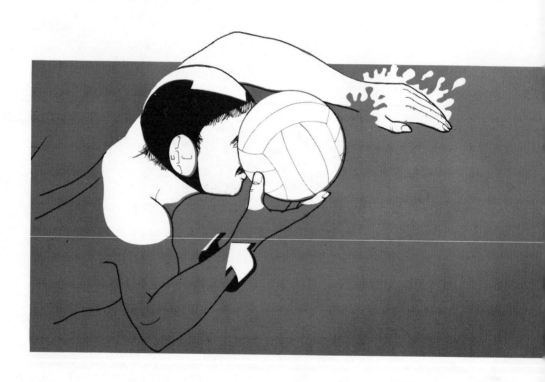

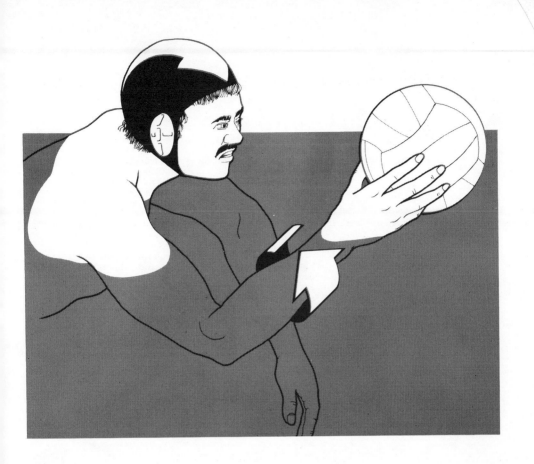

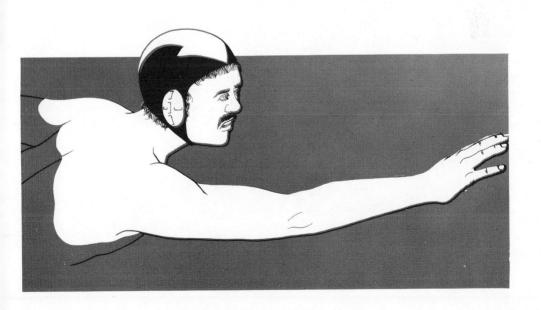

Memory Aid: Increase kick — arm tempo — splash — hand under ball — cork-screw.

PROBLEM	CAUSE	CORRECTION
1. Ball is consistently shot wild.	1. Your hand is flat against the ball, subsequently the ball rolls off your hand during the shot.	1. The ball should be held from underneath, supported equally by your five fingers and making minimal contact with your palm.
2. Ball is shot directly into goalie's stomach.	2. Too close for the shot.	2. Don't shoot closer than three meters.
3. No power on the shot.	3. Two possibilities: a) your hand is not pulled back far enough; b) you're not twisting your arm through the complete 180 degrees.	3. a) You should pull back your hand with the ball toward your head and almost touch your nose with the ball. b) The cork-screw effect must be one smooth motion, your arm twisting throughout the shot, not just at the beginning.
4. Ball is plowed right into the water.	4. You have just pushed the ball from behind.	4. Start with your hand cupped under the ball.

POP-SHOT

1. Your guard is close to your hips. You have the ball and are between three and five meters from the opponent's cage.
2. Accelerate your kick and shorten your stroke. Use a sloppy hand entry to set up some splash.
3. As your hand enters the water for a stroke pick up the ball from underneath on your fingertips. Lift the ball just high enough to clear the water. Make sure you don't toss the ball into the air but keep it on your fingers like a golf ball on a golf tee.

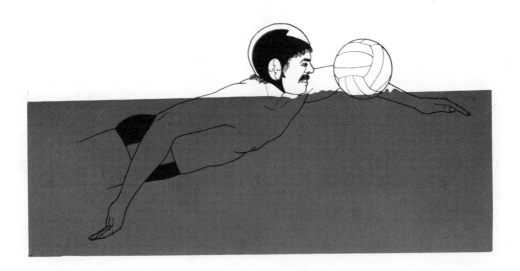

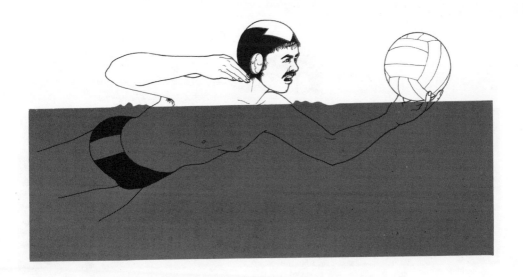

4. Your free hand should just be finishing its stroke. As it returns, keep your elbow high. Drive your hand toward the ball, your fingers pointed at the ball.

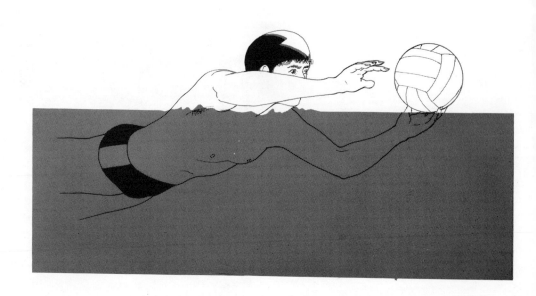

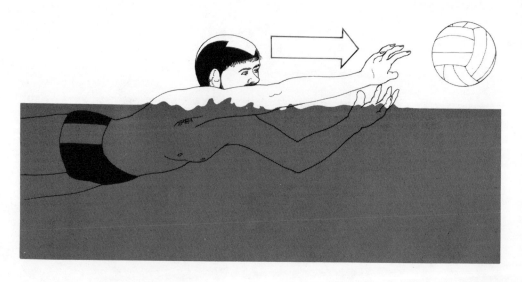

5. Look at that spot on the ball that you intend to hit and never take your eyes off of it. The major mistake made by most players is to look at the cage at this stage of the shot. You should pick your corner earlier. When you are in this close the shot and its direction are totally dependent upon where you strike the ball. Once again, look at the ball, not at the net.

6. Drive your hand into the ball at an angle so that the ball is directed at a corner of the cage.

Memory Aid: Kick — shorten stroke — splash — tee-hand — look at the ball — hit with pointed fingers.

Variation: Instead of maintaining the ball on your tee-hand, toss it a foot into the air. Drive your shooting hand through under the ball with a definite splash. As the ball is coming back down, pull back your arm so that it lands on your palm, then proceed to do a cork-screw shot, pages 36-41.

PROBLEM	CAUSE	CORRECTION
1. Goalie seems to be prepared for your shot.	1. You are giving him advance warning by: a) stopping prior to shot; b) rising out of the water; c) lifting the ball high out of the water.	1. a) Keep your kick going throughout the shot to keep your momentum. b) Make sure your shoulders stay flat on the water. c) Raise ball out of water no higher than is necessary to clear the water.
2. Ball goes wild, never where you want it.	2. Your hand is striking the ball flat. The ball is given no direction and rolls off of the thrusting hand in any direction.	2. Point your fingers as if you were doing pushups on your finger tips. Strike the ball such that each finger makes equal contact.
3. You miss the ball when striking at it.	3. Two possibilities: a) you're not looking at the ball; b) you're throwing the ball into the air.	3. a) Keep your eye on the ball. b) Make sure that the ball rests on your tee-hand.
4. You consistently hit the goalie in the stomach.	4. You are waiting too long to take the shot and have gotten too close.	4. Shoot between three and five meters.

REAR-BACK (RB)

The RB is most effective when there are too many defensive men in front of you, or when your guard seems to be concentrating on stopping your drive.

1. The situation when this move is most often used is as follows: A man of your team has been fouled close to the opposing team's cage, 2 - 2½ meters, and has a free throw. Your guard is between you and the cage.

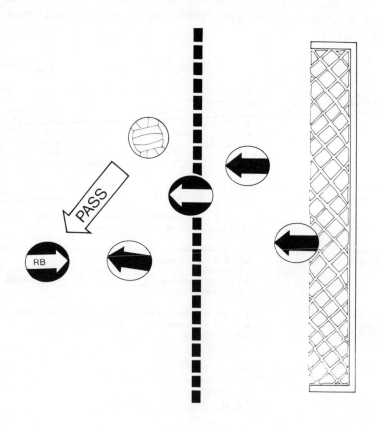

2. As your teammate picks up the ball to make a pass start your move.

3. Hips high, lift the arm out of the water that you intend to shoot with, and thrust it forward as if you were about to drive. It's important to look as though you are going to drive to put your opponent off-guard.

4. Instead of taking a stroke, push down on the water with a slap and raise your hand for the ball.

5. As you raise your hand, roll to your side and scull vigorously with your free hand.

6. Your legs should quickly be drawn under you and commence a furious egg-beater to get as high as possible.

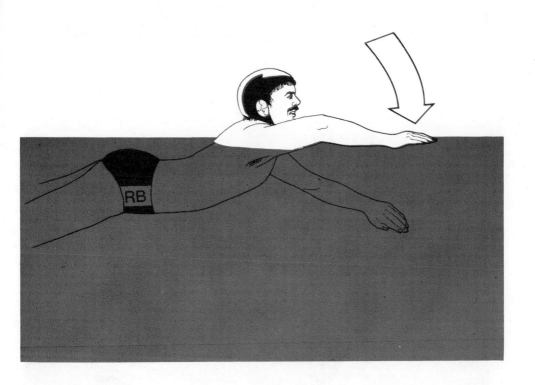

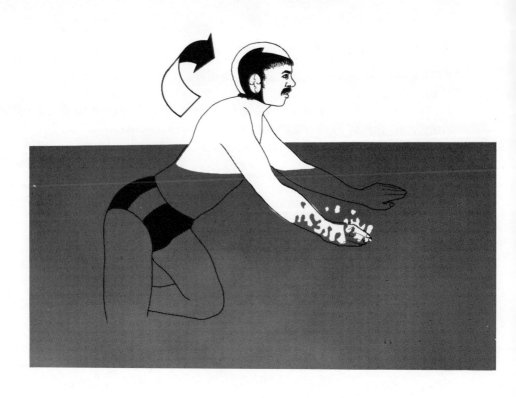

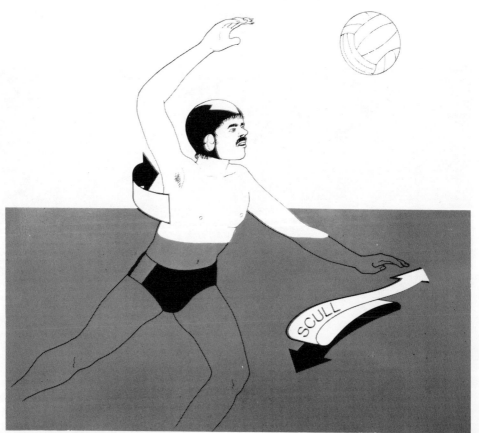

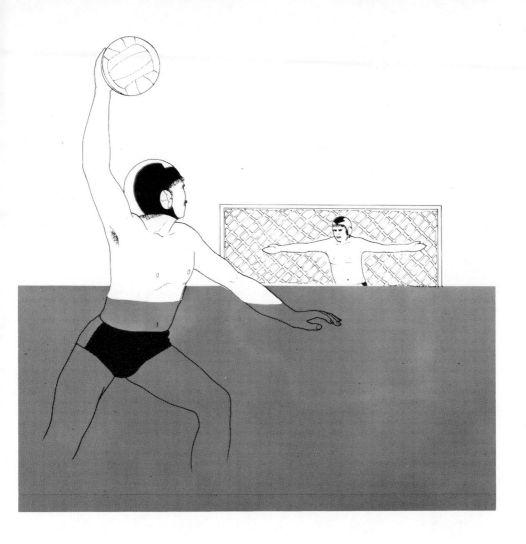

7. The pass must be quick, hard, and accurate, as you have less than one or two seconds to shoot the ball.

Memory Aid: Fake stroke — raise arm — roll and scull — egg-beater — shoot.

PROBLEM	CAUSE	CORRECTION
1. Shot consistently goes high over cage or has little power behind it.	1. You are laying on your back for the shot, a poor position for most shots.	1. Lean forward, supporting yourself with your free hand.
2. The hole man throws the ball in the water where you were driving, rather than to the RB.	2. You were probably beating your man and the hole man expected a drive.	2. Never RB when beating your opponent.
3. Your guard consistently knocks the ball from your hand as you receive it.	3. You have merely slowed down for the move.	3. Come to an abrupt stop.
4. It seems to take a long time to get the shot off after receiving the ball.	4. The pass has little power behind it, and you are forced to carry the ball back rather than shooting it forward.	4. The passer must throw the ball almost as hard as a shot, so the ball's momentum carries your arm back into shooting position.
5. You are consistently called for a pushoff foul.	5. Your free hand was used to push a guard away.	5. Your free hand should be used to brake with and for sculling.

FORWARD FAKE

Many players make the mistake of trying to grip the ball and pump it when making a fake. The method described here can be very convincing.

1. Rise high in the water with an egg-beater kick.
2. Start the move as if you were taking a regular shot.
3. As your arm is nearing its full extension, rotate your wrist so that your hand goes in front of the ball. This will act as a brake and keep possession of the ball.
4. This fake should start to the outside of your body. The ball will take a curving path and finish almost directly in front of your face.

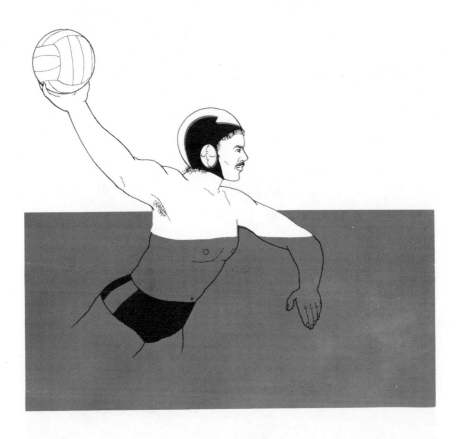

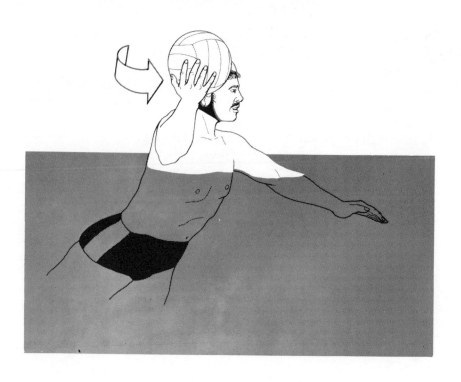

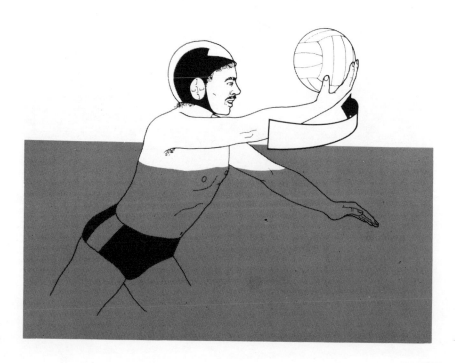

PROBLEM	CAUSE	CORRECTION
1. Goalie never rises to your fake.	1. Not convincing.	1. Look at the goal as if you intend to shoot; many goalies read eyes. Rotate your shoulders just as you would do in a real shot.
2. Ball fumbled and dropped.	2. You have either extended your arm too far or have failed to rotate your hand behind the ball.	2. More of a circular motion on the fake will make it easier to maintain possession of the ball.

BACK-DOOR KICK OFF

This is one of the highest-scoring moves in water polo.
1. Swim next to your opponent and slightly ahead. Your guard is between you and the ball.

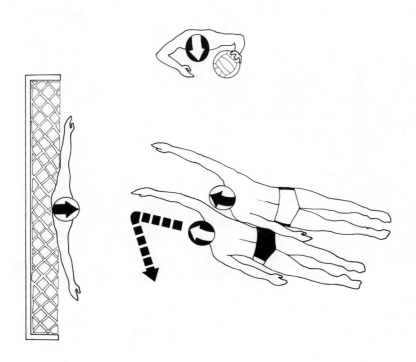

2. As you reach the three- to five-meter area in front of the cage, plant the top of your foot against your opponent's hip.

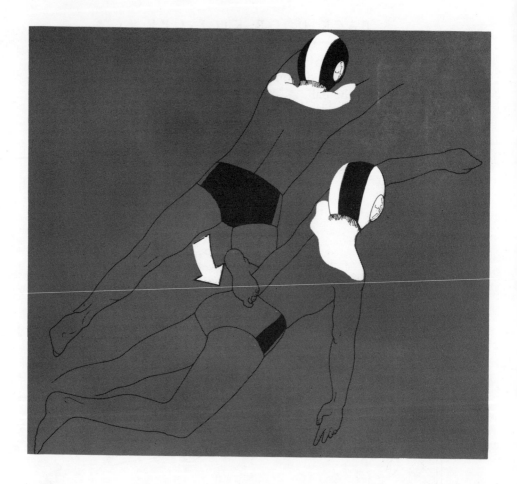

3. Now push away from your guard while maintaining your freestyle stroke.

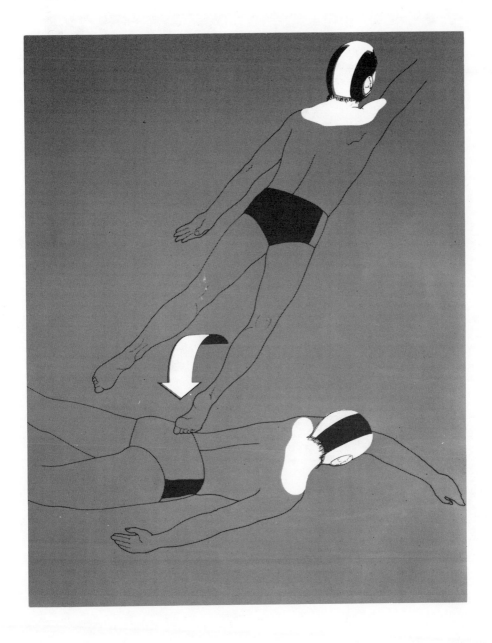

4. Roll to your back such that your shooting arm is free of the water and ready for a quick, dry pass.
5. I recommend that you roll away from, rather than towards, the cage.

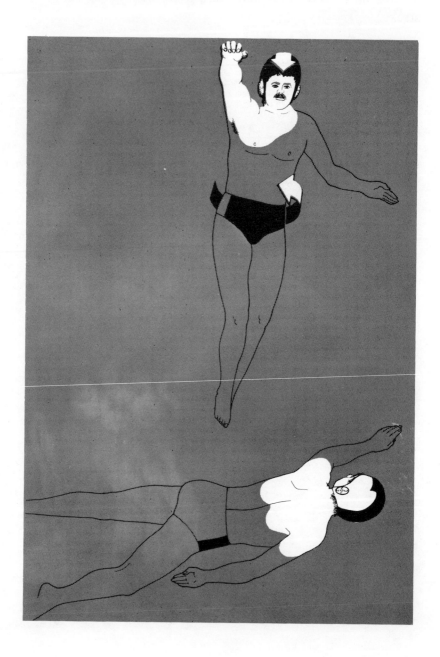

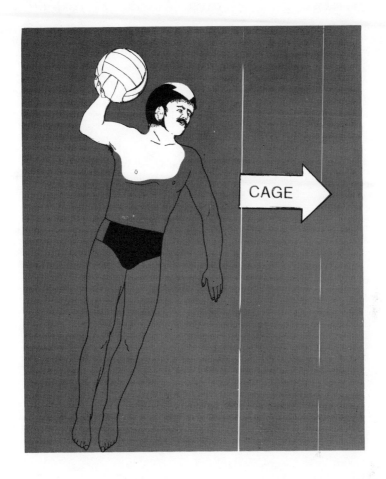

CAGE

6. If the goalie lunges for the side you have rolled to then shoot to the far side of the cage. If the goalie maintains a relatively central position then shoot for the near low corner.

Memory Aid: Lead — plant foot to hip — push — roll to backstroke — shoot.

PROBLEM	CAUSE	CORRECTION
1. Pushoff is ineffectual and opponent is right with you.	1. You have probably pushed off against the man's thighs or legs.	1. Make sure your foot is right above the hip bone and that it doesn't slip.
2. You are repeatedly called for fouling.	2. One of two problems: a) rather than pushing, you are kicking the opponent; b) you are rolling to your back for the push. Referees are alert for this type of kickoff.	2. a) Plant your foot, then push. b) Stay on your stomach in freestyle position throughout the pushoff.
3. Difficulty in catching the ball. Your shooting hand is often underwater when the pass comes.	3. Arm cycle is too slow when on your back.	3. Increase your back-stroke arm cycle, taking short, rapid strokes.
4. When you finally receive the ball you are some distance from the cage in a small pool, maybe even touching the side wall. You have a poor angle from which to shoot.	4. You have swum down the pool in a line with the post and then pushed off toward the near wall.	4. Try to swim down the center of the pool or slightly to one side so that when you push off you end up in line with a post on the cage.

3 Defensive Pass Blocking

CHEST-BLOCK STRAIGHT ARM

This defensive position is done in order to block a pass or force an error. It also prevents the player from going immediately and tires him. Too often players in this position get excited and foul. Remember that it is much harder for your opponent to make a good pass when you put nonfouling pressure on him, rather than giving him a free throw.

1. Opponent has ball and you are guarding from behind. Keep both hands up with your arms on either side of the player. Use a powerful egg-beater, hips high, constant pressure against man's back.

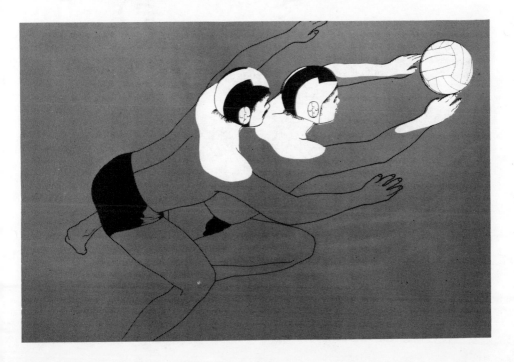

2. As he rolls to his back to pass, place one hand on his chest. This pressure forces your opponent down, and he must either pass immediately or roll to his stomach. (This concept of *rushing* the pass is basic and forces the other team to make errors.)

3. Raise your other hand straight up in the air to block the pass. Preferably, if he is passing with his right hand, raise your left hand to block and place the right hand on his chest.

4. Powerful egg-beater to raise your body.

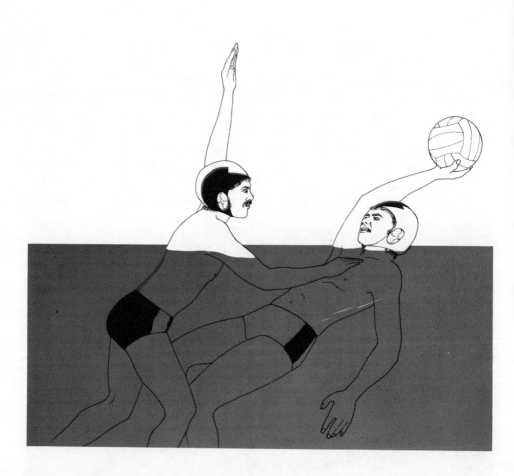

5. Do not become overly excited at the sight of the ball. The moment the opponent puts the ball down go back to your guarding position in number 1. Many players swim right over the opponent for an unnecessary foul, which gives the man a free uninhibited pass with little chance for error.

6. Raising your arm straight up is usually better than reaching for the ball (unless your opponent makes the mistake of putting it too close to his head). The reason for a straight arm is that if he passes, it must be high enough to clear the arm and, subsequently, fairly slow and inaccurate.

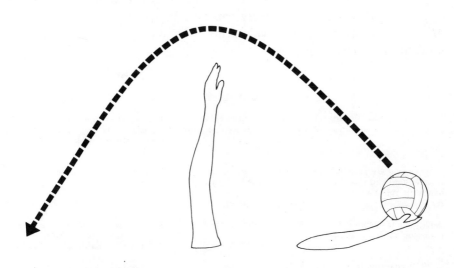

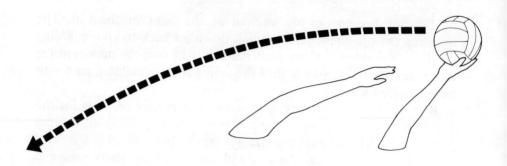

7. If he manages to make the pass, then give him a forceful push underwater with the hand you have on his chest. Most referees will follow the ball down the pool and will miss this foul. This tires the passer and if used consistently can take its toll by the third quarter. *Memory Aid:* Hands out — wide arms — hand to chest — blocking arm straight up — push him down.

PROBLEM	CAUSE	CORRECTION
1. Opponent consistently gets away to make a good pass.	1. You are not keeping constant pressure against your opponent's back.	1. Keep your hips high to prevent a pushoff and egg-beater constantly. Don't be shy about contact.
2. When you are guarding from behind and have both hands up, referee calls you for fouling.	2. You are resting your elbows on the man's back or are gripping him with your elbows.	2. Keep your arms wide, forming a U.
3. Opponent pushes off from you and then makes pass.	3. Your hips are low.	3. Your bathing suit should be no more than an inch below the water in guarding position.
4. While guarding from behind opponent wraps his legs around you.	4. Probably because your hips were down.	4. Two options are available when this problem occurs: a) raising your knees vigorously will cause the opponent to unwrap his legs; b) without his legs your opponent has no way of maintaining his station, and you can move him towards a wall or fellow player.

CHUGGING

This can be a very infuriating defensive maneuver. Its purpose is to force a player driving down the center of the pool to move to the side where his potential usefulness is diminished.

1. Face your opponent with your hips up. It's best to be less than an arm's length from your opponent. This situation is common just after a foul has been committed by someone else or at halfway after a goal.

2. Angle your body to one side to give the man a way to go. Preferably force the man towards his weaker shooting side (i.e., when facing a right-hander, with your cage behind you, force him to your left). Do the opposite for a left-hander.

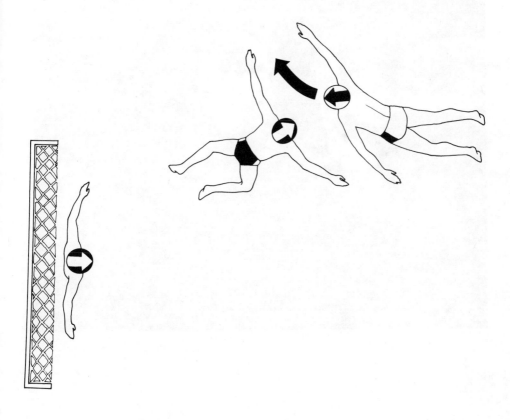

3. As the player approaches give him a *guiding push* in the direction you want him to go. Make sure you hit his chest, not his head, shoulders, or neck. Alo make sure you are pushing to the side not straight back.

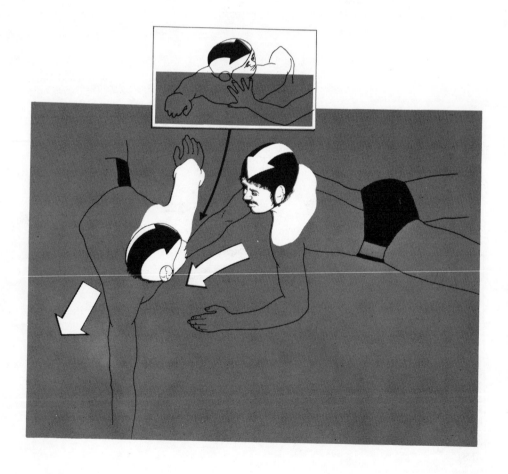

4. After one or two guiding chugs, turn with your man shoulder to shoulder and swim with him. Don't let him get in front or in back of you. Now funnel him towards the wall.

5. When he's near the wall take the pressure off.

6. The most powerful use of chugging is during the faceoff when the other team has the ball. Each of your teammates calls out a number so no one is missed.

7. Chugging will slow down their drive and give your sprinter a chance to get through to the man who has the ball. The passer will be forced to put the ball down, and this will keep the ball in their half of the pool with less chance for them to score.

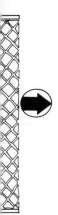
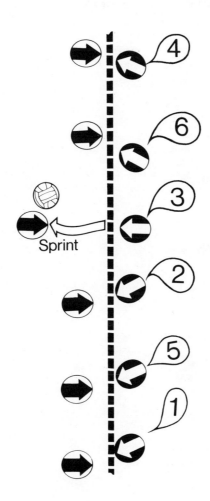
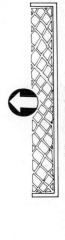

Memory Aid: Arm's lenth — angle — chug — swim and funnel.

PROBLEM	CAUSE	CORRECTION
1. Referee calls you for fouling.	1. You are doing one of two things: a) chugging too high out of the water; b) or chugging straight on which forces him up out of the water.	1. Keep chugging on the chest. Give him a way to go and push him there, preferably the weaker side.
2. Opponent always seems to get by.	2. You are giving him a chance to develop too much momentum.	2. Get closer before he starts swimming.
3. As you chug or push the player he grabs your wrist and pulls by you.	3. You're giving a long slow push.	3. A chug should be just as the name implies — a quick piston-action push.

4 Offensive Passing

COUNTER TO A
CHEST-BLOCK STRAIGHT ARM

1. You have just passed the ball and the man defending you has tried to block the pass by putting one hand on your chest and raising his other arm straight up.
2. Assuming you have made a good pass, rather than being pushed underwater by his weight, use his momentum against him.
3. Grab the wrist of the hand on your chest and pull the hand off your body toward his opposite side. Next, give a slight downward tug.
4. His own momentum will carry him down, and you will be able to swim by him.

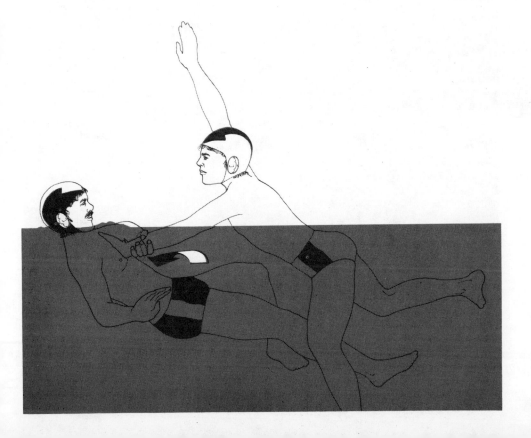

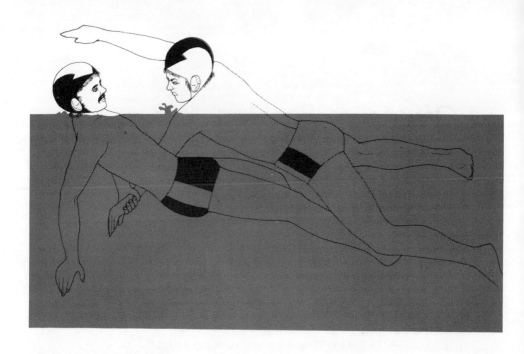

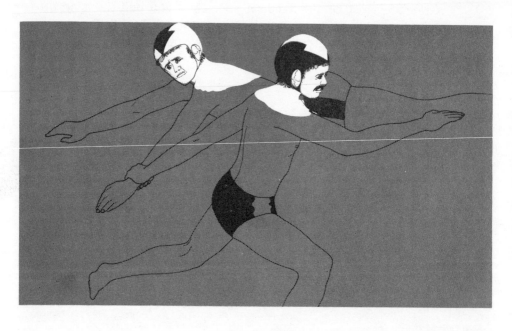

5. This move usually catches your opponent off-guard as after a pass most players stop for a moment; only a mentally tough player goes immediately after a pass.

Memory Aid: Grab wrist — pull to opposite side — pull down — go.

PROBLEM	CAUSE	CORRECTION
1. Rather than going to your side the man goes right down into you.	1. You are pulling his hand down to the wrong side of your body.	1. If his right hand is on your chest, pull it toward his left side.
2. You pull his wrist across but just can't seem to get going.	2. Player has pushed you down too deep, making it difficult to get started.	2. Make your move sooner, before you are scraping the bottom of the pool.

CROSS-CHICKEN LEG

When you have the ball and are guarded from behind this will get you enough room to roll and pass.

1. Opponent is guarding you from behind.

2. Bend your left leg at a ninety-degree angle and cross it over the back of your right leg. Your left foot should now be near his right hip.

3. Curl the top of your left foot around his right hip. It's important that your foot be curled around just above the hipbone as you have your best leverage there.

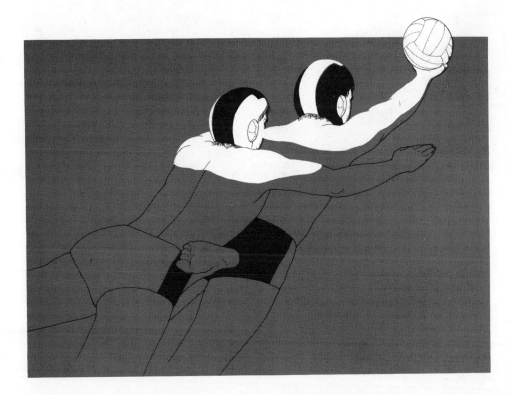

4. Now in a forceful motion, pull your crossed leg, the one on his hip, back toward its normal position. This should push the opponent to the outside of your legs.

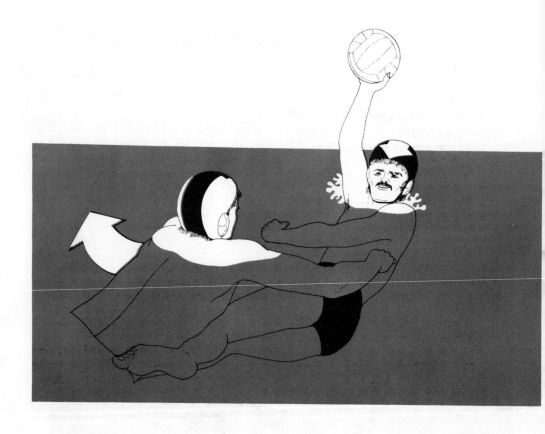

5. As you push player to outside of your legs, roll to your back with ball in your hand ready to pass. The roll, if the push is done with the left leg, should lift your left shoulder out of the water.

Memory Aid: Ninety-degree angle—foot on opposite hip — push — roll facing — pass.

PROBLEM	CAUSE	CORRECTION
1. Pushoff is ineffectual and guard is still tight on you.	1. You have failed to hook his hip and have slipped when you pushed, or you have pushed against his legs.	1. Your foot should form a shepherd's crook, which fits right above the hip of the guard.
2. As you roll, your legs get tangled up and you can't push.	2. You have rolled the wrong way.	2. The roll, if done left-footed, should enable you to see the man. Don't roll so that you lose sight of him momentarily.
3. Ball is knocked from your hand.	3. You have held ball too close to your head where he can reach it.	3. Hold ball at full extension behind head.
4. Guard seems to be prepared for the move.	4. You have probably put a hand on top of the ball, signalling you are about to try something.	4. Pick up ball from underneath.

5 The Hole Man: Shots and Defense

SHOULDER-IN

This is a hole man's shot, and it takes advantage of the length of your arm combined with your shoulders in order to get a shot at the cage.

1. Position yourself in front of the cage, ideally right on the two-meter line. If you get pushed out to four meters your chances for a hole shot go down. Position yourself such that you are centered in front of the cage.

2. Keep your arms wide to prevent opponent from slipping in front of you. They should be right at the surface ready for the move.

3. Your opponent's position must be somewhat vertical in the water.

4. Pick up the ball from underneath so as to give the man guarding you the least amount of time to prepare for your maneuver.

5. Pivot rapidly so your shoulder is put into your opponent's chest, with the ball held at full extension.

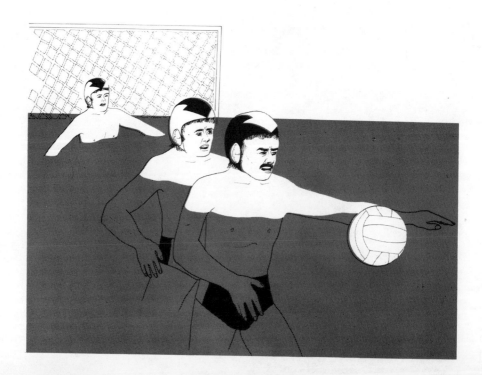

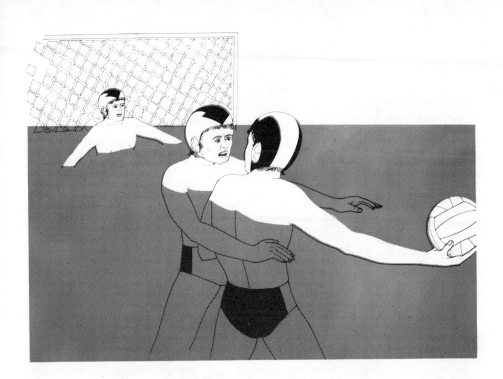

6. You should egg-beater vigorously and take care not to push the guard away with your free hand, as this would be an offensive foul.

7. With the length of your shoulders and arms combined it is unlikely that the guard will be able to reach the ball or get a decent grip on your arm, and you will have some time to shoot.

8. If you feel the guard starting to go over you, then either put the ball down or shoot. The first alternative will usually get the guard called for fouling as he cannot react quickly enough to get off you.

Memory Aid: Ball from under — pivot shoulder in — scull — shoot.

PROBLEM	CAUSE	CORRECTION
1. You consistently lose ball via an underhand steal.	1. Ball is too close to your body, or possibly opponent has an exceptionally long reach.	1. Ball should be at arm's length, readily picked up from underneath, hips high.
2. Ball is hit from your hand after you get your shoulder in.	2. Holding the ball near your head.	2. Arm holding the ball should be fully extended behind you.
3. Referee calls you for pushing off.	3. Instead of putting your shoulder in, you are pushing off with your free hand.	3. Make sure you are sculling with your free hand.

CLAMP

When set in the hole position, your guard will often try to make an underhand steal. This move allows you to take advantage of his tactic and possibly discourage him from trying it again.

1. Player reaches under your arm to steal the ball.

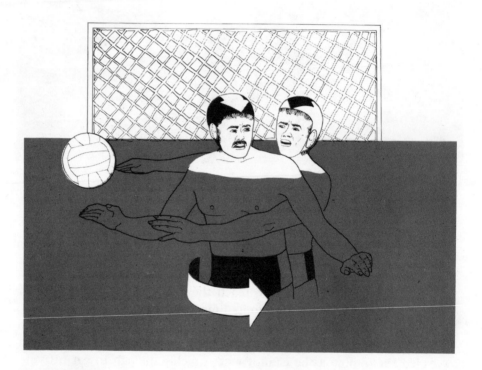

2. Clamp his arm, preferably his bicep, directly under your armpit.
3. While gripping his arm in the clamp, pick up the ball from underneath with your opposite hand. Pivot against his arm. When you pivot, rotate in a tight position against your opponent's body. Don't pull away or you'll lose him.
4. After the pivot you should be facing the cage with the ball in front of you and your opponent behind.

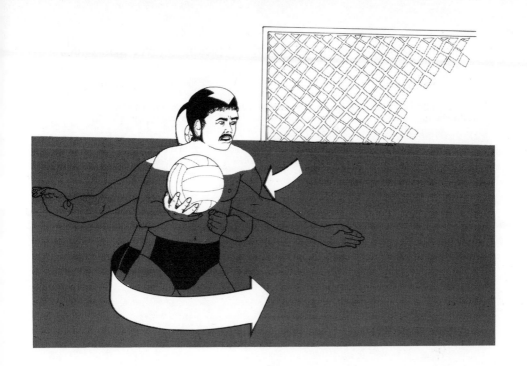

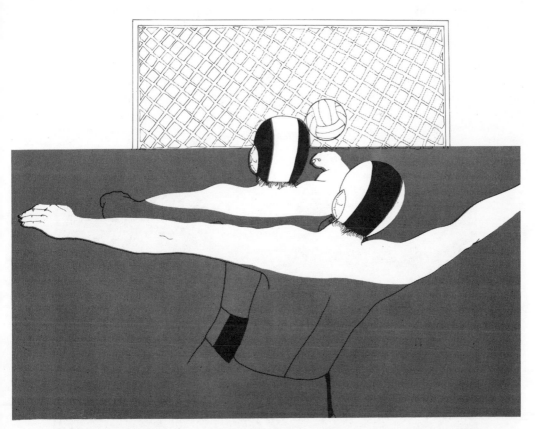

73

Memory Aid: Clamp armpit — underhand pickup — pivot tight circle.

PROBLEM	CAUSE	CORRECTION
1. Man continually pulls free of the clamp.	1. You are clamping his arm too low against the side of your body.	1. Dip down a little to get his arm under your armpit.
2. Instead of turning him you go up over his shoulder for a foul against you.	2. You're not staying in tight against the man.	2. Make sure he is against your back. Don't pull away as you make the move.
3. He winds his legs around you in a desperate attempt to stop you.	3. This is a mistake on his part; don't stop turning.	3. By wrapping his legs around you he has lost any means of preventing your spin. This is to your advantage; just egg-beater harder.
4. You seem to pivot right into the man guarding you so that you are face to face.	4. You pivoted the wrong way.	4. If his left arm is clamped under your left arm, pivot to your left.

STRAIGHT-ARM PIVOT

1. You are set in the hole and have possession of the ball. The man guarding you drops his hips. Pick up the ball from *underneath.*
2. Take your free hand (usually your left hand if you are right-handed) and place it on your opponent's hip. Straighten your arm out and keep it rigid. It's important that you lock all the joints on your arm until it's as stiff as a two-by-four. Now pivot your body like a child's top.

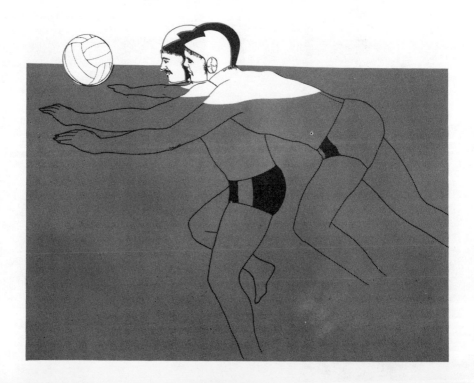

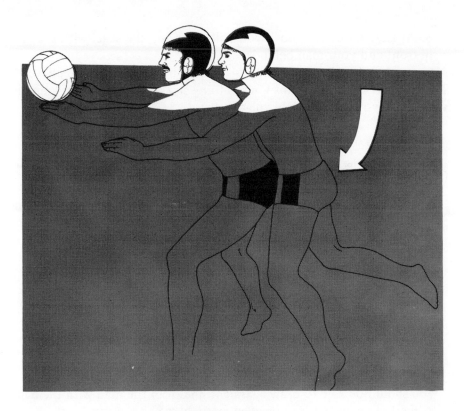

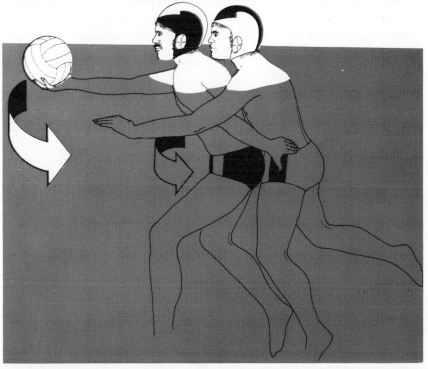

3. At the end of the move you will be facing the cage, with the ball in front and your man behind.

Memory Aid: Hand to hip — rigid — pick up ball underneath — pivot.

Variation: If the guard grabs your bathing suit, reach down and grab his wrist. With your arm straight, pivot.

PROBLEM	CAUSE	CORRECTION
1. Referee calls you for a pushoff foul	1. You are pushing guard away or down with your straight arm.	1. Once you place your hand on the guard's hip, you use the force of your pivoting body to bring him around.
2. You continually lose the man.	2. You are reaching for him.	2. Opponent should be firmly against your back.
3. You turn right into the man; he hasn't been moved at all.	3. Your arm wasn't rigid.	3. Your shoulder joint is probably the one that moved.

GUARDING THE HOLE MAN FROM IN FRONT

This is the first of two basic ways to guard the hole man.

1. Position yourself in front of the hole man.

2. You should be directly between him and the man with the ball. You should be able to draw a straight line from the man with the ball to the hole man, with yourself directly between the two on the line.

3. Face the hole man with your hips high and no more than a half an arm's length away. It's best to have one of your shoulders pointing at the hole man and the other at the position where the ball is.

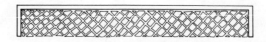

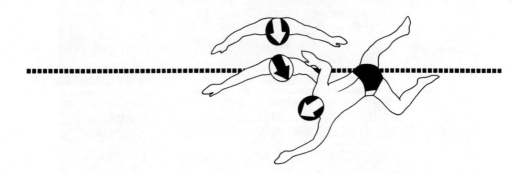

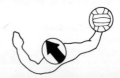

4. The most important thing in this position is that you always know where the ball is. Your head should be moving like a lighthouse beam.

5. If the goalie comes out just a little, you can sandwich the holeman and make it extremely difficult for him to get the ball.

6. As long as the hole man is in the four-meter area you can guard from in front when the ball is outside. As the hole man moves over four meters you should guard from behind. This has served your purpose, as you have forced the hole man out of the scoring area.

PROBLEM	CAUSE	CORRECTION
1. Hole man pushes off from you and gets pass for shot.	1. You either have your back to the man and he is using it like a platform from which to push off, or your hips are down.	1. Face man with your hips up.
2. Man consistently gets passes, and you don't seem to be able to block them.	2. You are not directly between ball and man or are further than an arm's length away.	2. Put yourself between ball and hole man an arm's length or less away from the man.
3. Ball is passed over you to hole man who scores.	3. Either goalie is not coming out enough or you have moved out beyond four meters.	3. Tell goalie to move out a little, or move between hole man and cage.
4. Ball comes in and shot is taken before you can do anything.	4. You don't see ball coming.	4. Turn your head rapidly keeping an eye on the ball.

GUARDING THE HOLE MAN FROM BEHIND

1. First rule is to keep your hips up with a strong egg-beater, pushing against the man.

2. Keep your chest against your opponent's back. Put your chin on his shoulder, preferably his shooting side. Putting your chin here is important, for it will give you some grip on your opponent; it also prevents him from developing any momentum if he intends to hit you with a backhand.

3. Your arms should cradle the man. A cradle is formed by holding your arms wide like the letter *U*. Keep your hands right at the surface, shadowing his arms.

4. As he attempts a shot, slap his wrist down or hold him at the elbow. This usually causes an ineffective shot, which the goalie can handle.

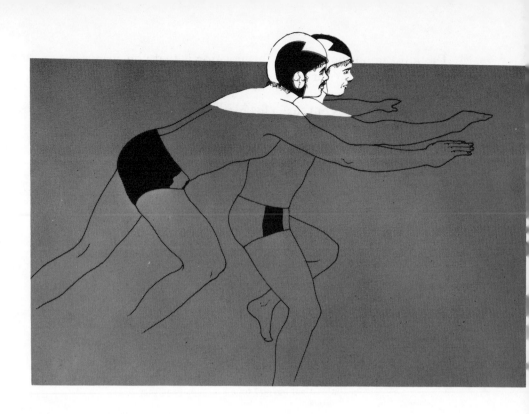

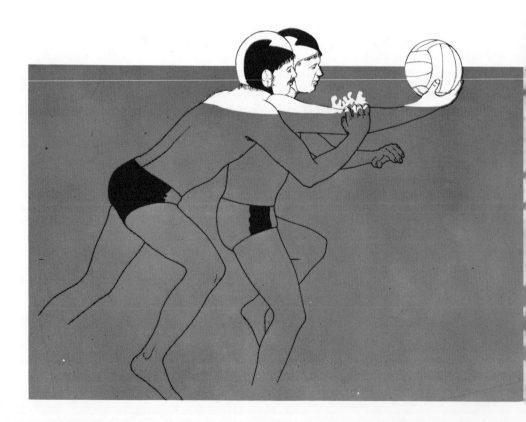

5. To frustrate the hole man you can splash water at the ball to move it out of his reach and force him to move away from the cage.

Memory Aid: Hips up — chin pressure — cradle — wrist or elbow.

PROBLEM	CAUSE	CORRECTION
1. Hole man gets his shoulder turned into you and gets a good shot off.	1. You are not providing constant pressure against the hole man's back.	1. Hips high with a strong pushing egg-beater.
2. Hole man gets off shot.	2. Your hands are not close enough to his arms.	2. Shadow the hole man's arms with your arms.
3. You get hit in the head with an arm during a backhand shot.	3. You are hesitant to make close contact.	3. Put your chin on opponent's shoulder.
4. You get your hand grabbed underwater.	4. Your hands are not being kept near the surface.	4. Break the grip with a counter to a wrist grab, pages 82-84.
5. It seems that the hole man has taken the shot, but too late you realize he still has the ball and he gets off an uncontested shot.	5. You have either: a) instinctively closed your eyes as he faked a shot; b) turned away from the player and probably looked at the cage as a fake started.	5. Some hole men will make what appears to be a threatening backhand shot to prompt the guard to close his eyes. If you keep your head near his head you are not likely to be hit and will not close your eyes so readily.

UNDERHAND STEAL

This maneuver is used to steal the ball without fouling. It is very effective when a player can be pushed up against the wall and has little room to work the ball.

1. You are guarding an opposing player from behind. He has the ball but allows it to get too close to his head. There are two ways to effect a steal:

2. Reach under the arm of your opponent and, using a wrist flick, flip the ball over his head.

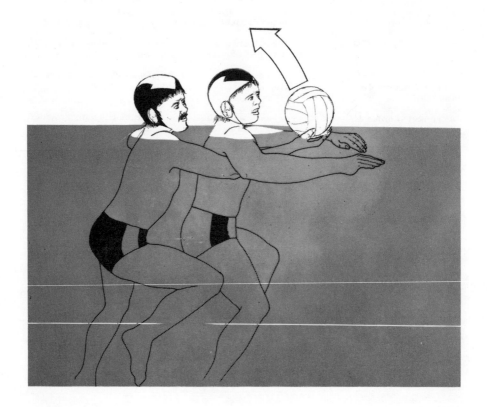

3. You should now have control of the ball.

4. Another method can be used if the ball is slightly out of reach:

5. Start with your hips high in the water. Reach under his arm (your left under his left, or vice versa). Scissors kick forward as you roll to the side. Your roll should be a complete 360-degree spin. This lunge should allow you to reach the ball and flip it in front of your face.

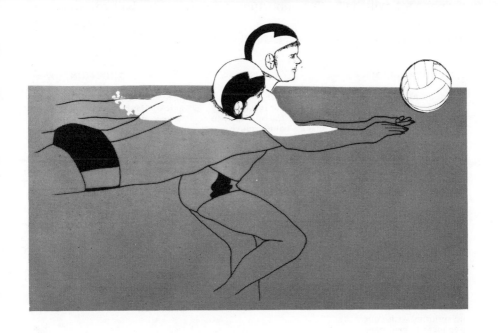

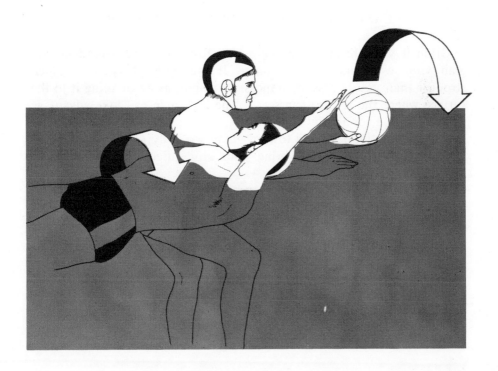

6. This is a somewhat risky move, for if you fail to get the ball your opponent will have the opportunity to swim the ball toward your cage.

Memory Aid: Reach — scissors — roll — flip.

PROBLEM	CAUSE	CORRECTION
1. Opponent clamps your arm under his and turns you.	1. You are slow and hesitant in your reach, giving time for the opponent to make a countermove.	1. Reach forward smoothly and quickly. Make sure you don't leave your arm out too long.
2. When going for a long reach with a spin you consistently miss the ball, and your opponent is left free to swim at your cage.	2. The man you're guarding is probably baiting you — tempting you with the ball.	2. Watch his hands; see if he keeps them close to the ball when moving it within your reach.
3. Continually called for fouling.	3. a) You are reaching over his arm. b) You take so much time that the referee may assume you are fouling.	3. a) Reach under the arm. b) The flip must be one smooth, quick motion.
4. When doing an underhand steal with a spin you manage to flick the ball but usually end up sprinting with your opponent to gain possession.	4. You have tossed the ball directly in front of you.	4. The flick should put the ball on the far side of your body away from your opponent.

COUNTER TO A WRIST GRAB

Often if you are guarding the center forward from behind he will grab your wrist and hold it under. If the center forward is much stronger than you it may be impossible to pull away or bring it to the surface where the referee can see it. The hole man can take advantage of this position for a number of shots.

1. Pull your trapped hand toward your own body.

2. In a twisting motion bring your arm quickly up behind your opponent's back.

3. In essence you now have an arm-lock, and most hole men will be quick to realize their vulnerability and will release your wrist. If they don't let go you can exert more pressure until they are made aware of their predicament.

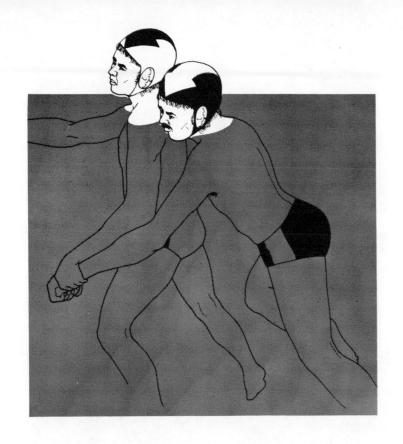

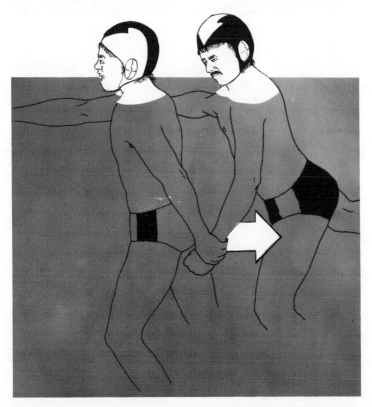

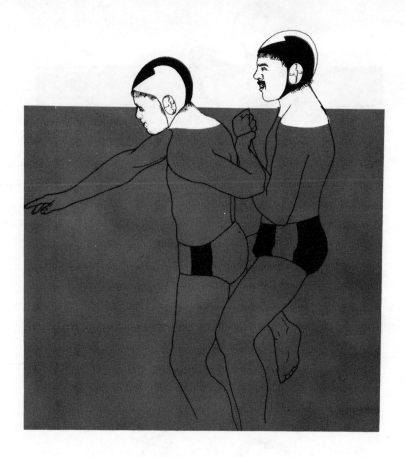

PROBLEM	CAUSE	CORRECTION
1. Can't twist your arm up behind opponent.	1. You probably haven't pulled your arm towards your own body.	1. To get the proper leverage you must pull his hand behind him.
2. Hole man grabs your wrist and immediately shoots the ball.	2. The quickness of this type of move is hard to counteract.	2. Immediately reach over the hole man's shoulder and blatantly foul him. It's more important to prevent his shot. Just don't let your hands get caught underwater again.

6 Tips

1. Many of the moves described in this book depend upon the element of surprise. If your opponent is wary, you can set him up to be surprised in the following manner: Make convincing stunts and feints as if you were going to drive at the cage. Force your opponent to keep his eyes riveted on you. After awhile he will probably begin to wonder what is going on in the rest of the pool. This is when you take advantage of him. Relax for a moment as if you've given up hope of driving. At this moment your opponent usually turns his head to see what is going on. When his head is turned he is offering his hands for wrist grabs, hip rolls are easy, or just sprinting past him is now possible.

I often have to remind my players that they are being snake-charmed. Snake-charming is the art of forcing your opponent to watch you so intently he loses track of the rest of the game. I've seen numerous situations where the player is so concerned with the man he's guarding that he fails to notice a ball directly behind his head. The best way to overcome this is to keep your head moving like a lighthouse with rapid glimpses rather than television stares.

2. Before attempting any maneuver that may be considered a foul, take a glance at the referee. Doing a move directly under the scrutiny of the referee is difficult unless you are an expert. And try to remember that referees are not omnipotent, and they can make mistakes. They do not usually make these mistakes on purpose, but your shouted abuse, looks to kill, or gestures can tempt them to want to see you at a disadvantage. Remember they are as human as you are.

3. Keep your hips high when on defense. Many players are hurt or are

responsible for an opposing team's goal because they were vertical in the water. It's just too easy to kick a player when his hips are down. One of the quickest ways to tell a good player from a bad one is to watch what happens when the referee blows the whistle for a foul. A poor player thinks of the whistle as rest time and drops his hips, if they aren't already down.

4. If you have problems with other players using your bathing suit like a luggage handle, try the following: Purchase one of the new three-ply water-polo suits. These suits fit much tighter and, because of their cut, are more difficult to grab.

To restrict grabbing even more, try winding tape around the top of your suit and part of your body. This prevents anyone from reaching into and holding onto the suit. As a suggestion, make sure the player takes a deep breath while winding the tape around his suit so it will not constrict his breathing.

5. Many players shy away from mouthguards. The mouthguard has more advantages than just preventing broken teeth, and it does not restrict your breathing — a common misconception. If you are not worried about losing your teeth you can play a more aggressive game. And where one player without a mouthguard would be decked by an elbow under the chin, the protected player would be able to keep playing and maybe even return the favor. Wear a mouthguard.

6. When wearing a water-polo cap with long string ties, never make the mistake of leaving a dangling string. I've seen players grab these loose strings or a large bow and pull their opponent's head underwater, and maybe give a kick or two to the fettered player. Always wrap any loose ends carefully around the chin strap.

Index